DIY: Reflexology

*A Beginner's Guide to Reflexology
for Pain Reduction, Stress Relief,
More Energy, Health and
Wellness*

By Bryan Thompson

Bryan Thompson

Bryan Thompson

The information provided herein is stated to be truthful and consistent, in that any liability, in terms of inattention or otherwise, by any usage or abuse of any policies, processes, or directions contained within is the solitary and utter responsibility of the recipient reader. Under no circumstances will any legal responsibility or blame be held against the publisher for any reparation, damages, or monetary loss due to the information herein, either directly or indirectly.

Respective authors own all copyrights not held by the publisher.

The information herein is offered for informational purposes solely, and is universal as so. The presentation of the information is without contract or any type of guarantee assurance.

The trademarks that are used are without any consent, and the publication of the trademark is without permission or backing by the trademark owner. All trademarks and brands within this book are for clarifying purposes only and are the owned by the owners themselves, not affiliated with this document.

Discretion: I am just a passionate student of health & wellness and am looking for the most cutting edge strategies that can benefit my life, which inspires me to share this knowledge to anyone willing to listen.

Author's Note: I realize that my words will not resonate with every reader. As a man committed to constant and never-ending improvement, if you have any <u>constructive feedback</u> that you would like to offer, or feel like the content in my book can be <u>improved</u> in any way...

...please feel free to contact me at:

faithinknowledge@bookenthuziast.com

Table of Contents

Introduction

Reflexology is an ancient and alternative medical art that can address even modern aches and problems. Aside from being non-invasive, the techniques in this book can be done in the comfort of your own home and without the help of a hired professional. Aside from the cost and time savings you get from reflexology, learning how to *do it for yourself* will also prepare you when you plan to do it for your loved ones who may need it in the future.

This book gives you a brief overview of the principles behind reflexology, such as the flow of qi, the reflex zones and the pressure needed for the sessions. These principles are then translated into specific and practical techniques that can address common and modern conditions of the body.

This book teaches you about reflexology techniques for the following conditions:

1. Muscle tension

2. Stomach discomfort

3. Stress

4. Headaches and migraines

5. Sleep disturbances

6. Toxins

7. Coughs and colds

8. Asthma

9. Hypertension

10. Eye tension

11. Diabetes

12. Menstrual pain

13. Skin disorders

14. UTI

15. Weight Loss

The techniques in this book can also be practiced *without prior training*, making it ideal for use even for beginners who aspire to learn and to use an alternative form of medicine.

Plus, a primer on everything you need to know to jumpstart your pursuit of excellence in reflexology is added in this book. General hand, foot and face techniques are shared with you so you can learn to use reflexology not only as a therapeutic exercise but also as a preventive solution to health risks.

A background of reflexology, such as its history, schools and the different tools and supplies will give you an appreciation of the progress and developments that reflexology has undergone to become one of the most popular alternative health methods of the modern day. While reflexology is effective as it is, when used in conjunction with other similar alternative health treatments, then its potency becomes enhanced. Acupressure, acupuncture and other techniques are also discussed to show your options on how to make a better and more holistic program for your use.

This book will also share you tips on how to select your reflexologists. While reflexology can indeed be done on your own, there will be cases when you many prefer or require a professional to assist you. To help you make the best decision, visiting local and online resources, conducting due diligence and estimating average cost of sessions will also be discussed.

Also, you will learn how to manage your expectations on reflexology. This book will give you information on what to expect before, during and after a session in reflexology. It will give you an idea on the limitations of reflexology, such as health situations that contraindicate its use. Finally, information will also be shared on further studies on reflexology should you become interested in pursuing advance knowledge of this worthwhile endeavor.

Begin your journey towards self-healing! Use reflexology today!

Bryan Thompson

Chapter 1

Basic Principles of Reflexology

The practice of reflexology has various techniques, styles and applications. In fact, aside from the traditional applications, new techniques are being developed on a regular basis. This is because the ever-changing stresses and demands of the human body in the modern day require reflexologists to adapt and cater to their patients' health needs. Still, whether traditional or modern, each technique is developed and built using three of reflexology's main principles.

These principles are:

1. Meridian point

2. Qi and energy flow

3. Acupressure

Qi & Energy Flow

Qi, popularly known as chi, is the natural energy that flows in every living being. The concept is primarily Chinese in origin and it is also the basis of other Chinese medical and martial arts. Reflexology relies heavily on the concept of qi.

Those who believe in qi suggest that this form of energy flows and permeates into every part of our bodies. A free-flowing and balanced qi is able to keep the body and mind healthy and in prime condition. The better the flow of your qi, the healthier you are and the longer your life can be.

On the other hand, physical or psychological trauma, injuries or other factors can affect this flow. When the flow is disrupted or blocked, the imbalance is manifested in the form of physical symptoms. Therefore, in reflexology it is not only important to treat the actual symptoms of the illness but also to correct the imbalance.

Reflex Zones

To correct the flow, reflexologists rely on specific locations in our body, called reflex zones. While acupuncturists use meridian points, a reflexologist uses a chart that divides the body into ten zones. The point of reference can be found on the feet, specifically on the soles, divided by your ten toes.

Imagine four lines that start from the space in between each toe on your left and another four lines on your toes on your right foot. In between those lines, you have five spaces. Now stand on your feet with your feet flat on the ground. Now, imagine those spaces in the sole of your feet extending all the way up to your legs, thighs, torso, arms, shoulders, neck and head. These are the zones of reflexology that cover your entire body.

The idea behind the treatment is that every symptom that can be traced to a specific organ of your body can be addressed by locating that same organ on the zone where it belongs. For example, when a qi disruption occurs in the liver, which is on the right side of the body, reflexology treatment will also be done on the right sole in and around the zone which the liver belongs to.

For more specific treatments, reflexologists also developed the concept of the five lateral zones on top of the ten horizontal zones. To find these five zones, sit in front of a mirror and raise your feet so that you can see the reflection of your soles. Now look at the entire length of your toes, this is the zone of your head and neck. The line that separates the toes with the rest of the soles of your feet is the zone of your shoulders.

Next, look find the balls of your feet, these are marked by a bone on each of your foot that slightly protrudes, forming a mountain-like structure in your sole. If you cannot find it, try reaching the soles with your palms and press it gently until you find the bones. When you found it, the space in between the shoulder line and the edge of bottom edge of the bones is the chest zone. The actual edge of the chest zone, the ridge of the bones is the zone that is connected to the diaphragm or the muscle that is responsible for our breathing.

Next, find the bone on the bottom part of your feet; this should be a solid and flat bone where the heels of your shoes would be. When you find it, the gap in between the diaphragm line and this flat bone is your abdomen zone, the lower border of this zone is connected to the pelvic area of your body. The last area of on your soles is the lower abdomen zone. Aside from the soles of your feet, you can also find reflexology zones on the palms of your hands.

Bryan Thompson

Often, beginner and even some expert reflexologists will need a chart to help them locate and remember the reflex zones. Here are some links to resources that can provide you with these charts.

1. Hand Reflex Chart:

   http://www.distanthealer.co.uk/reflexology_study_chart s_colour.htm

2. Feet Reflex Chart: http://reflexology-map.com/feet-map/

Take note that you will come across charts that present the reflex zones in slightly different areas. This does not necessarily mean that one chart is wrong and the other one is correct. These charts only present the general areas on how one organ in the body is connected to a specific spot either in the feet or hands.

Also, aside from only the feet and hands, there are other reflex zones scattered in the body that you can use.

Knowledge of these basic zones are very important, especially for do it yourself reflexology sessions. Aside from knowing the general area that you need to focus on, you can also engage in preventative measures when you are known to be at risk for developing certain illnesses.

Pressure

Now that you know the causes of the symptoms and the specific zones that you need to focus on, the actual method of applying pressure on the zones needs to be learned. Although there is no hard and fast rule on the style or intensity of the pressure, most reflexologists use firm pressure on the reflexology zones. Take note as long as you can use your hands to generate enough pressure on the zones that is all that is required.

The idea behind reflexology is that the nerves found in the soles of the feet and the palms of the hands are all connected to the central nervous system of the brain. When you massage the zones, you also stimulate these nerves, which in turn trigger the release of chemicals, like endorphins, in the brain that can produce beneficial effects. For example, endorphins act as natural pain killers that lessen the pain or act as relaxants that relieve stress.

Take note of your pain thresholds when you apply pressure. Use only your fingers and thumbs for your reflexology sessions. Test your limits, when you find the right pressure that is just below being painful, then that is the correct pressure.

If you are unable to use your fingers for some reason, like arthritis, wounds or anything that will make you unable to create enough pressure for the zones, then you can use reflexology instruments. They can be purchased from various alternative medicine stores, such as Eastern medicine pharmacies. However, some are expensive. If you are on a budget, you can make use of household items that can produce the same results. For example instead of purchasing a feet roller, you can use a golf ball or any similarly shaped object to roll on your feet.

Bryan Thompson

Chapter 2

DIY Reflexology on the Feet

Prep Work

There is really no prescribed or special preparatory work before any reflexology session. As long as you are calm and comfortable, you can begin anytime. Most reflexologists suggest sitting in the flat surface, preferably a yoga mat, with your legs crossed. Wear comfortable clothes and loose pants so that you can sit comfortable and you will not constrict any movement. Consider washing your feet first with warm to lukewarm water.

Applying scents, such as mint and other fragrances are not necessary but if they add to your relaxation, then go ahead. Oil can also be used, use just enough to allow your fingers to slide gently on your foot. Too much at your fingers may slip and prevent you from applying enough pressure. This is why professional reflexologists prefer not to use oils altogether. If you are a beginner, it is best to use oil in the meantime while you hone your skills. Others prefer soothing music, such as the sounds of flowing water or a slow melody.

Try to minimize if not, completely remove, any distractions such a loud noise or people who can walk past you during your sessions. However, if you are not bothered by these distractions, you can go ahead with your session. Try to find out and create your personal ideal environment that best suit you need for calm and comfort.

Muscle Tension

Reflexology Zone: Neck zone of the feet

One of the muscle groups that always suffer from tensions or stiffness are the muscles in the shoulder. This is primarily caused by sitting for long periods of time without the proper back support. Most office employees will have these problems.

Begin by applying pressure on the neck zone of the feet. You may start from the interior side of your foot and then all the way to exterior side. Once you reach the exterior side, give particular attention to the area below your smallest toe. If you look the soles of your feet, the skin in this area should noticeably be darker than the rest of your soles. Apply pressure on this area.

If you have a feet roller, you can use it to generate enough pressure on this area. If not, you can substitute any round object and use the palm of your hands to roll the ball back and forth on the area.

Bryan Thompson

Take note that if you have muscle tension on your shoulders, expect this area to be very sensitive. Do not immediately apply pressure or use the roller, instead begin with gentle touches and explore your pain levels.

You can also use this technique on other zones on your feet if the muscle tension is elsewhere. For example, if you have back pain, then the location is the middle strip of your sole. This strip can be found starting from your middle toe all the way down to your heel bone. This imaginary line also represents your back and your spine. Once you reach the midway on this line, apply more pressure.

Stomach Discomfort

Reflexology Zone: Abdomen zone of the feet

Another modern problem caused by artificial and unhealthy diets is stomach discomfort. There may be reflux, ulcers, gas, constipation and other discomforts in the digestive system. Use these two reflexology techniques to address these set of problems.

First, locate the abdomen zone of the feet and from there you can determine the general area where your diaphragm and pelvic zones are. Next, use your forefinger and your middle finger. Use a walking motion with these two fingers, this can be achieved by pretending that the two fingers are your legs and you will walk on the lines of these zones. Now walk your fingers on the area between the diaphragm and pelvic zone. It may be ticklish at first but you will get used to it. As you walk your fingers, you need to apply more and more pressure and reduce the level of pressure when it becomes painful. This technique targets your stomach and intestines.

The second technique can be done by putting pressure on another site on your feet. Instead of the sole, you need to look at the back side of the sole. Locate the gap in between your big toe and the second toe. From this ridge, bring your finger around an inch below that point. Apply pressure and gently massage this area. This technique targets your abdomen.

Stress

Reflexology Zone: All ten toes of your feet.

The daily stressors in life, especially in the modern age, can potentially take its toll on the well-being of anyone. Stress can affect your physical, psychological, professional and social statuses in life. Since stress is for the most part developed and felt in the mind, all ten toes of your feet, especially the two big toes will be your zones for this therapy.

Apply firm pressure on the sole-side of your toes. Most reflexologists use a pinching technique. Put each toe in between your thumb and your pointing finger and press them together. Apply pressure for about a minute, beginning from a light and progressing to heavier pressure until before you feel pain. Do this for all the toes. Extend the duration of the pressure on your big toes. The toes are very sensitive to pain but with the right pressure, it will trigger the release of endorphins in your brain to create that calming effect you need to relieve your stress.

Bryan Thompson

Chapter 3

DIY Reflexology on the Hands

Prep Work

Instead of sitting on the floor, the prep work for hand reflexology needs you to sit in a chair. Choose a spot that can also create calm and comfort for you. Clean your hands thoroughly with lukewarm water and soap. If you are a beginner, it is best to use any hand lotion that you may already have at home. Allow 2 to 3 minutes to coat and massage your hands with the lotion. Wait until all the lotion is absorbed by your hands to prevent slipping.

Since the palms of your hands are more sensitive than the soles of your feet, doing hand reflexology has an additional benefit. As you massage your hands, take note of any feeling that is out of the ordinary. For example, it could be a spot in your palm that feels tender, harder or softer than usual when you press on it. You may also feel a crunch when you press a spot for the first time. When you spot these areas, try your best to remember where it is. You can either mark it with a pen or hold on to the spot while you refer to a reflexology chart.

Since the palms also have reflexology zones, these abnormal spots in your palms may indicate a disturbance in the flow of your energy. With exact spot, you can even go further to detect on which organ the disruption is present. Through this detection, hand reflexology can act both as a therapy and as a diagnostic tool.

Other prep work involves cutting your nails so they will not press on your skin. Make sure that you schedule your hand reflexology session before sleep or when you do not expect to make use of your hands in a couple of hours. While some want to avoid washing their hands after a session because it will cause tremors, there seem to be no medical basis for massage causing tremors.

Finally, if you have arthritis, pain or any abnormal condition on your hands, reflexology for your hands is discouraged. If this is the case, you need to rely on other body zones to relieve yourself from the illnesses.

Headaches & Migraines

Reflexology Zone: Four sides of all your fingers

Migraines are becoming more and more prevalent today and it is a condition that is not only painful but also inconvenient. The pain is so great that some people are unable to proceed with their normal daily routine. This technique is meant to be used as quick and easy way to relieve the pain as soon as the condition strikes.

Bryan Thompson

The pinching technique, similar to the one used on your foot for stress, will also be applied in this therapy. The only difference is that you will spend more time and more attention not only the front and back side of your fingers but also the sides.

Use all your right four fingers to support the base of each left finger. Using your right thumb, apply pressure on your left thumb. Start with tip of your thumb on the fingernail side of your finger. Press gently in one pressure level for an entire minute. Next, rotate your finger and now press on the left side of your thumb and continue pressing as you move downward to your wrist. With those two steps, you should have been able to press on all four sides of the thumb. Do this for the remaining 9 fingers.

Another technique that you can use is to apply pressure in the most sensitive spot in your palm. This can be found on the gap in between your thumb and forefinger. Pinch on this area, with your opposite forefinger on your palm and your thumb on the backside of your palm. Press as hard as you can and release the pressure before it becomes painful; remember to take deep breaths in between the release.

Sleep Disturbances

Reflexology Zone: Thumb

Insomnia, inability to achieve a deep sleep and other sleep disturbances are also health issues. Adequate rest, provided only by a complete and relaxing sleep, is necessary to rest both your mind and body to make it ready for next day's work.

Before you sleep, find the exact center of your thumb, most can find it on the point where their fingerprint swirls. Now, use your opposite thumb and turn it to its side, you will use the side corner of your nail for this technique. Rub the side of your nail to the center of your thumb. Do this for a minute.

Toxins

Reflexology Zone: Liver zone of your palm

Without discipline on your diet, not only will digestive problems occur but also toxins will be retained on your body. In small quantities, these harmful chemicals can be processed and filtered out to your system by your digestive organs. However, when toxins increase in levels, the digestive system, especially the liver, may be unable to filter them out effectively.

Find the liver zone of your palm, since the liver is on the right side of your body, you will be using your left hand to apply pressure. Find the spot by tracing a straight line from your pinky finger. When you reach 1 inch below the base of the pinky finger, move your finger to the right and press gently as you go along. You will feel that the area becomes softer with the middle area softest. Stop when you reach 1 inch below the base of your thumb. The wide area you just traced is your liver area.

Massage this area using your left thumb. Make sure to avoid pressing too much as the area in the center will be very sensitive. Spend about 5 minutes in this massage. When you are done, turn your focus towards the other side of your palm. Using the same direction in tracing the liver on your palm, you can find your liver zone on the other side.

Once you are done, it is best that you drink around 2 to 3 glasses of water. Once your liver is relaxed and the toxins are filtered out, you can help out in the detox process by adding liquids in your body. Take note every time you use reflexology therapies that are meant to detoxify your body or that will involve your digestive organs, conclude your sessions with a glass of water.

Bryan Thompson

Chapter 4

DIY Reflexology for Common Illnesses

Aside from the hands and feet, there are other points that you can massage to create relief and restore the proper flow of your qi. Take advantage of your ability to reach these points to address some common illnesses.

Coughs & Colds

Right in the middle of the area where your neck meets with your shoulder line is the point that you need for to address coughs and colds. When you press it, you should feel that it is hollow. If you found the right spot, then apply pressure with your forefinger. Do this for 3 minutes. Aside from coughs and colds, this point can also address other associated illnesses such as heart burns, sore throats and congestions.

After this, move your fingers down from the hollow area and to the side. You are looking for the area underneath the breastbone. When you press it, your fingers should slide upwards towards the other side of your breastbone. When you found it, apply enough pressure to keep your fingers on the desired spot.

Asthma

Around 3 inches below your collarbone are the two points you need to look for in this technique. To find this spot, begin by tracing your collarbone working your way towards the middle. You will feel the collar bone on both sides reaching an end when you near the bottom part of your neck. From this edge, go down

3 inches and you will have found the two points. Using your middle and forefinger apply pressure on these two points. You can alternate between the points using one hand or you can also apply pressure simultaneously using both hands.

Another location that you can use for asthma relief can be found on the base of your thumb. Face your palm towards you and locate the area where your thumb meets your palm. When you press it there should be a bone on the lower side and a soft spot on the upper side. Apply pressure on this spot for around 5 minutes. Be gentle with your pressure as this area is extremely sensitive to pain.

Hypertension

Face a mirror; you want to start in the point in between your eyebrows. When you found it, use your thumb and slide it all the way down to the tip of your nose. Use only one direction, downward, for this technique. Since the skin is very thin on this area, you need to use a drop of oil to avoid friction.

Eye Tension

For this therapy, you need to face a mirror again. Use your middle and forefinger and rest it on your eyebrows. When you are familiar with the spot, press gently and you should feel the bone that makes up the socket of your eyes. Make circular movements as you massage this area. Since this therapy brings your fingers close to your eyes, make sure that your fingers and hands are washed before the therapy.

Another common problem with eyes is redness often due to strain from prolonged use of watching TV and computer screens. The spot you need to pres is the area right below your eyebrows near your nose.

For clearer vision, allow your right hand to rest on your left palm. Rub both thumbs together for around 5 minutes.

Diabetes

Sit comfortably on a flat surface and move your legs and feet toward you bottom. On the leftmost side of your left leg, just below your knee you should feel a hollow area between the joints of your knee and the bone of your leg. Find the same spot on your right leg. Use your ring, middle and forefinger on your left hand for your left knee and your right hand for your right knee. Apply the pressure on these spots.

Menstrual Pain

Find the spot where your big toe meets the body of your foot. From this spot, move down around 2 to 3 inches, you should feel the bone that connects to your ankle. Now slide your fingers underneath this bone and apply pressure.

Bryan Thompson

Weight Loss

Stand in front of the mirror, you can either remove your shirt or wear something as light as possible. Find the last set of bones on the bottom of your ribcage. Apply pressure on both sides for 5 minutes.

Skin Disorders

You need to apply pressure on the bone that is directly below your big toe. It should be a bone that feels like a ball in your sole. Press the area of your right foot's ball; expect for it hurt a little if you are currently having skin problems. Massage the area in slow and circular motions. Do this for around 5 minutes. This spot is connected to your adrenal gland, also responsible for neutralizing skin disorders.

Another point that you can use can be found on your left palm. Move less than inch below the gap between your pinky and ring finger. When you press, you should feel two bones and a slight gap in between. Press this spot for about 2 minutes. This is the spot that connect your palm with your gall bladder. This organ is responsible for aiding digestion that will detoxify your body and remove wastes that affect your skin.

UTI

Sit comfortably on a chair. Choose a seat that will allow you to reach the back of your knees. Massage the backside of your knee. When you press this area, you should feel the soft spot that is in between two bones. Apply pressure for 5 minutes. Since this is a detoxifying therapy, remember to drink water after every session.

Bryan Thompson

Chapter 5

General Hand Techniques

Hand reflexology is the main go to technique for do it yourself reflexology. The advantage of these set of techniques is that you can do it on your own and anywhere, even at the comfort of your own home. This makes these techniques extremely effective and valuable for common pains that you need to relieve on your own. For example, complaints such as headaches, muscle pains and constipation are some of the health problems that can be addressed using general hand techniques.

However, despite the comfort and advantages of these techniques, hand reflexology still has its disadvantages. The reflex on the hands are much deeper compared to those in the feet, which are closer to the surface or the skin. This means that the effect of feet reflexology are much more immediate compared to hand reflexology. Still, for days when you are unable to sit back, remove your shoes and use face or foot techniques, then hand reflexology is your best option.

Also due to the depth of the points, hand techniques require added pressure and a longer duration when applying pressure. Use your finger, preferably the thumb, on your chosen reflex point on the hand. Move your thumb in a circular motion, remember do not lift your thumb or finger as you rotate. Apply pressure for up to 5 seconds. Continue to the next reflex point and repeat the process.

Thumb Walking

In thumb walking, this a general reflexology movement which keeps physical contact with the skin as you move from one reflex point to another. Pressure is applied throughout the walk. To do this, put your right palm on a flat surface with your palm facing the surface. Put your left palm on the top of the right hand, also with the palm facing downward. Your left palm should be in contact with the back of your right hand.

Position your left hand thumb so that it rests directly above the knuckle of your shortest finger. Next, push your thumb starting from the knuckle, and then move it towards the center of your palm. As you move bend your thumb up then slide it down, as if like a worm inching itself. Make sure that every time you bend your thumb, the entire surface of the thumb gives contact to the skin beneath. Time your movement well, you need around 3 seconds with the thumb in full contact and applying pressure on the skin and then another 3 seconds bent and moving toward the next inch. Use this position to practice on the thumb walking technique.

As you familiarize yourself with this technique, you can pay attention on the finer points of the movement. You can make sure that your timing is correct, that the pressure you apply is sufficient and then you can focus on using the thumb walking to bring your fingers from one reflex to another. Remember, control is vital here, do not hasten the technique or make erratic rhythm.

Rotation

Another general technique is called rotation. In this movement, you again use your thumb but instead of sliding the surface of your thumb from one point to another like with thumb walking, you use the tip and you rotate in just one point. To do this, clasp all your fingers, except the thumb, inside your palm. Extend your thumb and point it downwards, the position of your palm should look like the "okay sign" but this time turned upside down.

To do the rotation, choose a point and rest the tip of your thumb directly above it. Divide three full rotations within a minute or 60 seconds. As you rotate the tip of your thumb, make sure that you press deeper and deeper with every rotation. Take note that as you perform this drilling motion, you make yourself flexible so that every rotation follows the contours of the muscle and bones beneath. Allow your thumb to shift instead of forcing itself to follow a perfectly vertical motion. Once you have finished with the minute of rotation you can continue with the next reflex point.

Take note, for this technique, you need to pay attention to hygiene. Make sure that your fingernails especially that of your thumb must be trimmed well. There has to be no sharp or uneven edges that can either scratch or scrape the skin when rotating. If needed, you can dab oil on the tip so that you can avoid friction when rotating. If you have an extremely sensitive skin, one that gets easily irritated, this technique may irritate your skin. Use this technique sparingly or avoid it entirely it. Instead replace it with a milder technique such as thumb walking.

Overall Routine

Remember, reflexology can also be used not only as a therapeutic but also as a preventive exercise. You can perform an overall routine that targets all available reflexes in the hand. Start with your right then the left hand. Begin by going into a relaxing phase. Rub the wrist of your right hand and massage towards the center of the palm. Do this for 30 seconds. Next, use your thumbs to apply pressure on the bottom side of each finger and your knuckles. Next, pinch your fingers and sway them from one side to another, do this gently. As you swing, maintain a rotational movement.

Next apply pressure or use any of the techniques discussed above on the meridians of the hand. These are found on both sides of the where the fingernails meet the flesh of the finger. Do one finger for 5 seconds. Next, apply pressure on the rest of the fingers. You need to start from the base of one finger, to the top and then move on to the next. Make sure that all sides, including the webbing in between fingers are massaged.

Next, rest your palm on a flat surface. With the palm facing upwards, massage the outer edges, the then the sides, and then the center of the palm. Remember to massage all the surface area of the palm. Turn your hand, this time massage the back of your palm. Start from the knuckles all the way down to the wrist. When done, do the same techniques for the left hand.

Finally, make sure to drink a glass of water immediately after the massage. Increase your fluid intake on the succeeding hours. This is because the reflex will have released toxins in your body and you need fluid to flush out these toxins more efficiently.

Bryan Thompson

Chapter 6

General Foot Techniques

The same principles of thumb walking and rotation apply for foot reflexology techniques. The only difference is that you have better access to the reflex points. This means you can apply gentler pressure or as much as you can tolerate but still gain access to the points. This is the most common area for the reflexology techniques and the feet have the greatest number of reflex points. This makes the foot one of the best areas to practice your reflexology skills.

Bryan Thompson

Spinal Areas

Start your foot reflexology just as you would your hand reflex, with a relaxation exercise. To relax your foot, you need to loosen your foot and prime it for the massage. You can do this by making slow but firm massages starting from your toes, the sole of your feet, the top side and all the way to the heels. Complete the massage for 30 seconds. Next using both hands, grasp one half of the spine of your foot with one hand and another hand for the other half. Gently twist the spine in opposite direction. Do this for another 30 seconds. Do this for the other foot.

With your feet relaxed, next you need to apply any of the techniques listed above to the specific areas on your feet. Start again with the right foot and then continue with the left. Begin with the spine, from the top beginning on the level of the toes all the way down to the heel side of the spine. Next apply your preferred technique sideways starting from the spine then to the opposite side of the foot. Do this until you have covered the entire foot.

Toe Rotation

Next are your toes. Begin with the biggest toe and work yourself to the smallest. Start by holding each toe firm at its base and then rotate it in circular movements. Give each toe a gentle tug forward to stretch it. Next release your hold on the base and then hold on to the second joint this time. Repeat the circular motion and the tug. Continue by apply pressure on the every meridian point in the foot, such as the area where the fingernails meet the flesh of the finger. There are reflex points on all toes except for the middle toe. Make sure that as you rotate or stretch each toe, you support it with one of your other hands.

Meridian Manipulation

Next is the chest area of your foot. This is where the base of the toes meets the heel all the way to one third of the foot. To find the chest area, you can search for the two knobs or bones below the toes. They should be just before the bridge of the foot. Massage the chest area and continue towards the bottom all the way to the pelvic area of your foot. The pelvic area is the bony area which makes up your heel.

Next is the opposite side of your foot or the one above your soles. Apply even gentler pressure on these parts as this is the most sensitive part of the foot. Begin your massage at the same area where you started on the sole. The chest area of your feet is the flesh right above the chest area of your sole. Next is the side of the arch and then finally the area opposite your ankle. This is the part where your lower leg meets your foot.

Chapter 7

General Face Techniques

The face is an uncommon but still effective location for reflexology sessions. The techniques are similar except that the pressure is now lighter due to the sensitivity of the face. Also, a corresponding chart is needed to locate the meridian points that correspond to your target organ. While face reflexology can be done for others, with proper posturing you can also do it for yourself. If you are a beginner and you are still unfamiliar with the meridians point in your face, it is best to sit or stand in front of a mirror and have a copy of the chart within your line of vision.

When you are ready, familiarize yourself with the meridian points while touching them as you study the chart. As you become proficient, you will soon be independent of the chart and then require only a mirror to do the face reflexology session.

Next you need to be as comfortable as you can. Make sure that the face and shoulders are supported. If you are doing for others, then you can either position yourself behind the recipient or have him lie down and stand near their head. If you are doing it for yourself, use a face mirror or any reflective surface to help you observe yourself as you do the session.

Point-to-point Stimulation

The basic movement needed for face reflexology is the rotation. As you apply pressure, make circular motions directly toward the meridian point of your choice. Duration of the pressure is approximately 60 seconds, with half of the time in a clockwise and the other half in a counterclockwise rotation.

In point to point stimulation, there is a recommended order in which you put pressure on each of the meridian points. Most of the points have a mirror pair on the other side of the face, for example your kidney meridian point, located in the inner corner of your right eye is also present in the inner corner of your left eye. Apply pressure on these points one at a time and not simultaneously.

Your starting point is your thyroid meridian, which are in your neck, near the two knobs that make up your collarbones. Next is for the intestines, which is right in the middle of your chin. This meridian point has no pair. Next is directly below your lower lip, this is the meridian point for the pancreas. On both corners of your lips, where your upper meets your lower lip is the meridian point for the lips.

The meridian point of your spleen is located on the depression just above your upper and below your nose. On the tip of your nose is the meridian point for the stomach. Below your

Bryan Thompson

cheekbones or approximately in the center of your cheeks are the lymph and liver meridian points. For addressing digestion issues, trace your cheekbones and apply pressure. On the outer corners of the eyes are your colon meridian points. Begin tapping from the outer all the way to the inner corner of the eye to reach the kidney meridian point. In the spot right in between your eyebrows is the meridian for the pituitary gland. This is also the same spot that you need to stimulate for health concerns regarding the reproductive system.

Using your fingers, try to locate the topmost edge and the centermost point of your forehead, these will be the locations of your mental capacities and nervous system meridians. Second to the last spot is the ears, pinch and pull down your earlobes and then up again for general body relief. The final meridian point around 2 to 3 inches away from the center of your chin is associated with your sex organs.

Relaxation Phase

As with other reflexology techniques, face reflex requires a preparatory relaxation phase to prime your face and body for the session. To begin this phase, simultaneously use both fingers from both hands to tap the area right below your eyes. Do this in an up and down motion and then continue to the next facial part. From the upper tip of your ears, down towards the earlobes and then all the way to the jaw line until you reach the chin is the direction you need to follow. Spend around 30 seconds focusing on your chin, then around the edges of your mouth until the cheeks of your face. Continue to your nose and use the bridge to reach the forehead, the eyebrows itself and rub from the inner to the outer corner of the eyebrows. Once you are done with the eyebrow, continue the movement all the way up to the forehead until your reach the hairline. Use gentle massage or pressure all throughout this relaxation phase.

Bryan Thompson

Use of Water

Drinking at least one glass of water immediately after a reflex session is an important final step in the reflexology process. Whether it is plain water or tea, the added fluids will help flush out whatever toxins have been released during the reflex sessions. In fact, it is a good idea to increase your water intake for the next 12 to 24 hours after your massage or reflexology. The more fluid you take, the easier it is for the body to excrete freed toxins and the better the benefits you gain from the actual session.

Chapter 8

History of Reflexology

Ancient Origins

While reflexology has only been introduced to the Western world in around the early 1900s, similar practices have been well documented in the ancient world. For example, therapy where the focus on healing was on the hands and feet were seen in ancient China and Egypt as far back as 4000 B.C. Depictions show of treatments being done in Egyptian tombs and reliefs. For example, in an ancient Egyptian tomb of a physician, a painting shows that the physician massages the toes of the feet and the fingers of the hand. While Egypt was considered to be the origin of the healing techniques, it was spread throughout the world via the expansion of the Roman Empire.

Fast forward to the early 1900s, the first version of modern reflexology is called the Zone Theory. William Fitzgerald, a medical doctor specializing in EENT, published a series of articles involving the subject that discusses the anesthetic effects of massage, which he called Zone Analgesia. Based on his studies, he discovered that whenever he applied pressure on the areas or zone where a medical complaint or injury is present, the effect was that of pain relief. Furthermore, aside from the reducing pain, it can also give relief to the actual cause of the complaint. His studies are documented in his book, "Relieving Pain at Home." This shows that even at that time, pain can be relieved at the comforts of your home and healing can be achieved through your own hands.

A colleague of Dr. Fitzgerald, Dr. Shelby Riley extended the foundations of reflexology. Dr. Riley combined the longitudinal zones that Dr. Fitzgerald developed with horizontal lines that bisect the body and provide more specific locations of the reflex points. Perhaps the greatest contribution on reflexology, built on the foundations set by the Dr. Fitzgerald and Dr. Riley, were made by Eunice Ingham, a physical therapist. Applying the Zone Theory, she found a pattern on the reflex points that were previously identified. Based on her treatment of hundred of foot patients, she discovered that each point in the foot corresponded with a specific organ in the body. Her book, "The Stories The Feet Can Tell" spread across the world and was even translated to several languages. It became the basis of the reflexes of the feet.

Modern Uses

Today, reflexology has exploded in the modern world with applications widely implemented in various individuals, objectives and settings. With the adverse effects of artificially produced medicines and treatments, health conscious individuals are now looking for alternatives that have fewer side effects and less prohibitive in terms of pricing. This alternative health method is now being practiced to provide both treatment and prevention with the objective of total wellness.

Reflexology is now being in various clinics and wellness centers. Patients in need of relief from pain, stress and other psychological issues go to the more natural and safer method provided by reflexology. Some of the many avenues that reflexology has found its place is in the office setting. For example, some companies offer reflexology sessions as perks along with other health benefits and coverage. An entire industry of spas, wellness clinics and centers prove to be a lucrative business, especially in business districts.

In the world of sports and athletics, reflexology also found its place among them. It will be common for sports-related injuries and treatment to include some if not all of the principles of reflexology. Even manicurists in salons also provide short but effective reflexology sessions. Even some health institutions, such as hospitals and schools, are participating at least studying the art and its potency.

Reflexology in the World

Today, reflexology has found its place not only in the Eastern countries that are said to be its origins but also in Western and the rest of the world. Aside from the US, the UK is another country with a robust presence of reflexology that offers opportunities to receive quality care or be a part of their group. The last week of September is also observed as the World Reflexology Week. This is a time when professional associations and schools initiate and implement awareness and advocacy campaigns.

Bryan Thompson

However, you also have to be very critical when you are planning to receive reflexology sessions elsewhere. Different countries have different regulations that monitor the practice of these techniques. Some countries have institutions in place that provide certification and oversee the standards and compliance of reflexologists and wellness centers. Other countries though are more lenient and some have virtually no governing body to promote and maintain its proper practice.

Chapter 9

Reflexology Branches

Western & Eastern

While the objectives of Western and Eastern schools of reflexology are relatively the same, there are notable differences between these two schools. This is important to note so that when you perform DIY reflexology sessions for yourself or for someone else, you need to be consistent in which school you will use. The differences between these schools make it necessary so that you do not duplicate your sessions or bring more harm than healing.

Bryan Thompson

For example, Eastern meridian points are very similar to Western reflex points. Upon closer scrutiny of points represented in Western and Eastern charts, you will notice very important differences. In Eastern schools, the heart point can be found below the ball of your foot, while in Western the point is on the ball of the foot. While in Eastern charts, the thyroid reflex point can be found on the ball of the foot, in Western charts, the point is actually on the big toe. Aside from the location, there are also differences on the wideness of the point, for example the organs such as the ovary for women and testes for men are much larger in their space covered in the foot compared to Western charts.

Another notable difference is the application of pressure in the points. Western techniques are slower and gentler but still firm. Reflexology sessions using the Western school are more concerned with providing relaxation. On the other hand, Eastern reflexology techniques have almost the complete opposite in characteristics. Pressure is more intense and vigorous. The objective is stimulation rather than relaxation. In fact, when the pressure applied to a point causes pain, instead of reducing the pressure, it is increased and prolonged. It is believed that this pain is an indicator that the blocked is removed and the flow is being restored.

The use of a dull wooden stick is very characteristic of Eastern schools while Western tools primarily use bare fingers, thumbs and occasionally knuckles. Sometimes, these sticks are made of crystal instead of wood.

It is to be noted that not one set of techniques is better than the other. Sometimes, you will require a Western style while sometimes an Eastern style. If you want to have relaxation from stress, fatigue or anxiety then you may prefer to use Western techniques. However, if you want to resolve health issues and do not mind the discomfort of a strenuous reflexology session, then the Eastern set of techniques can be for you.

Ayurvedic

This school is said to be the combination of Western and Easter schools of reflexology and its techniques. While it was developed in Australia, its roots can be traced to the Ayurvedic principles of India's medical philosophies. In Ayurvedic it is said that inside the body there is a constant flow of energies, which allow every cell and organ to function. This energy called prana courses through the body through a vast network of causeways or channels called nadis. The smoother the flow of prana within the nadis, the healthier the body and mind becomes. When the flow is interrupted or slowed, health issues arise.

The similarity with Ayurvedic and the Chinese concept of meridians becomes more apparent in the Ayurvedic concept of marma points. These are very important energy centers found in key areas along the nadis or causeways. These marma points ensure that the flow of prana is smooth. Similar to reflex points, the marma points are located in and the foot.

Ayurvedic reflexology encourages the use of oil as the lubricant of choice for its sessions. This is because any friction can only disrupt the very sensitive marma points. Typical sessions last for 45 minutes but the techniques are done very vigorously.

Rwo Shur

This is a school that is found mostly among Asian practitioners. It is said to have originated from a Swiss missionary in Taiwan. This is a unique set of techniques in reflexology because aside from using the thumbs and fingers to apply pressures, it also uses the knuckles and wooden sticks. Due to the hardness of the pressure, oil and cream are almost always used to avoid unnecessary friction. The pressure and motions are efficient and fast. Instead of relaxation, the objective of the sessions is to stimulate the reflex points.

Ingham

Named after Eunice Ingham, considered to be the Mother of modern reflexology, this technique revolved around the use of the thumb walking technique for reflexology sessions. Instead of targeted treatment, this is a more generalized or holistic approach to reflexology. Talc powder is the lubricant used for the Ingham method. The objective is to relax the body and achieve balance in the organ systems.

New Trends

The practice of reflexology is constantly being updated to address the growing and changing needs of the patients. The trend, especially in the West, is to augment reflexology sessions with techniques from other alternative medicinal approaches. For example, acupressure is being used as a reference for reflexology sessions. Other tools, aside from the fingers, are also being implemented to access the reflex points. Aside from oil and sticks, some practitioners make use of the magnets, and colored crystals are being included in reflexology sessions. Another trend is to surpass the limit of using only the feet and hands as points to massage. Today, ears are also being considered as a potential site for reflexology sessions.

Bryan Thompson

Chapter 10

Tools & Supplies

While Western reflexology only makes use of thumbs, fingers and sometimes knuckles, Eastern schools make use of an extensive set of tools and supplies to enhance each reflexology session. Take note that even if you are using Western styles or being attended to by a reflexologists using Western method, some of these tools and supplies may still be used.

Wooden Sticks, Rollers & Other Reflex Tools

The wooden stick is perhaps the most familiar tool being used in reflexology. While you can purchase these sticks online, there is nothing very special about them. If you prefer, you can make use of household items that have the same characteristics as a traditional wooden stick. Make sure that the stick has a dull or rounded point in the end to avoid piercing. Remember, in Eastern styles that focus is more on stimulation than relaxation. A wooden stick will be able to deliver more targeted pressure on your reflex point than your finger or thumb.

There are many advantages received on using the wooden stick. One is that it works faster and delivers benefits faster than using fingers. It gives you that much needed intensity that you cannot do when using your bare fingers alone. Uric acid that solidifies into crystals on your reflex points is usually shattered when you use these sticks, providing a brief feeling of pain but replaced by relief soon. When the uric acid crystals, which are the blocks to the proper flow of your energy, are removed, then your heath is restored.

Another tool being used in various wellness centers and being sold are wooden rollers. They come in various shapes and sizes. Generally, there are either cylindrical shaped rods or notched wheels that can provide wider areas of contact in one simple movement. Most are curved so that they follow the contours of every part of your body. Some are sturdy enough, like the foot rollers, so that you can put a portion of your body weight and roll your feet with greater pressure.

There other reflex tools that are used for either applying pressure or supporting the body during your reflex sessions. There are massage balls for the feet and hands, linens, foams, face rest pad and head pillows. One of the current best sellers is a thumb saver. This is similar to a thimble but with a curved tip that extends all the way to base of the thumb. This is meant to reduce the stress to your thumb as you put pressure in the reflex points without necessarily reducing the stimulation received by the reflex points.

Oils, Essential Oils & Aromatherapy

Another quintessential reflexology supply is the myriad of oils that are used either directly on the body or around the environment of the reflexology session. The aromas produced by these oils, aside from the lubrication, make them the perfect pair for every major objective of a reflexology session. Whether the goal is to achieve healing, promote wellness or alleviate other issues, oils are a welcome addition to your reflexology supplies.

Not all oils are made alike and each has their own therapeutic properties. The secret to maximizing their benefits is to find the oil that matches or enhances the goal of your reflexology. For example, if you want to be relaxed or gain relief from stress, then you can choose lavender, vanilla or rosemary oils and scents to enhance the relaxing effect of your massage. If you want to gain better control of your weight, then lemon, cinnamon and grapefruit are the best match.

Other oils will also have properties of their own. Oregano is an antibacterial essential oil, if you are using reflexology to promote recovery from infections, then this oil is your best choice. If a general detox is something that you are looking forward to for your reflexology sessions, then rose and juniper oils are your options. Reflexology sessions that target digestive disturbances, such as bloating or constipation, can be best addressed by cardamom. For skin issues, like acne or skin inflammation, you can use tea tree oil.

Take note that if you intend to use these oils, make sure that you follow the instructions of their use. Some oils are so potent that contact with the skin can cause significant irritation. This is why carrier oil is used along with main oil. The carrier is also another type of oil but is meant to dilute the potency of the oil so that it will be safe for use in the skin. Examples of carrier oils include olive, almond, aloe vera and sesame oil. If you intend to use these oils as part of an aromatherapy technique, to fill the room with the intended effects of the oil, then you need burners or diffusers. Remember to store these oils inside a brown glass bottles and away from direct sunlight to keep their effectiveness last longer.

Body Stones, Hot Bags & Other Warm Compresses

Usually used before or during reflexology sessions are various temperature altering tools that can prime the body, especially the muscles for more effective reflex massages. Body stones, which are soft, lightweight and highly heat absorbent and retentive rocks, are heated. They are then distributed and laid down on key points on the body, usually in the back and along the spine. The warmth of the rocks makes the muscles more pliant to kneading and reflexology techniques.

Hot bags are another alternative. Made popular in Thailand, these are small pillow-sized sacks that contain mostly grain.

These are then heated and the placed on the back and neck area. As with stones, they can be used over and over again. They are a better alternative to hot and cold packs because some sacks are packed not only with grain but also herbs for an added aromatic effect.

Bryan Thompson

Chapter 11

Reflexology & Other Techniques

Reflexology gives you an already very powerful set of techniques. However, when it is used in conjunction with other treatments, each of the techniques provides better results when complemented with other forms of alternative medicine. Perhaps, this is also the reason why reflexology is being confused with other techniques, such as acupuncture and acupressure. These two sets of techniques are said to have originated from the Chinese more than 5,000 years ago. An anecdote about the history of these techniques is that Chinese soldiers, who were pierced by arrows, reported relief from pain or sickness, which baffled court physicians.

There are several similarities and distinct differences between these therapies. However because they come from similar foundations they are two or three of them are used in one patient for a total session. Consider pairing your reflexology sessions with these other schools of alternative medicine.

With Acupuncture

A complementary therapy for reflexology is acupuncture. The basic principles of applying pressure and the specific points are very similar between these two treatments. However, the most obvious difference is that instead of thumbs or fingers performing the pressure, needles are being used. A very thin needle is inserted in specific acupuncture points that correspond to the health objective of the person.

The original purpose of acupuncture is to provide relief from pain but because of its many benefits, it is now being used in conjunction with reflexology for a more holistic experience. It can address allergies, digestive issues, weakened immune system, sleep disturbances, hormonal imbalances, blood and heart problems, weight control and also signs of aging.

If you intend to use acupuncture techniques, then make sure that it is being done by a trained, licensed or professionally recognized acupuncturist. Different people have different levels of pain tolerance, while some are able to tolerate the pain, some feel no pain at all and some are noticeably distressed with the insertion of the needle. Also the level of skill of the acupuncturists may also have an impact on the pain felt during the insertion. In reflexology, only the hands, feet and face are massaged but in acupuncture, needles can be inserted in almost any surface of the body.

Aside from physically inserting the needles, there are other ways to manipulate the needles to vary the effect of the acupuncture sessions. For example, needles can be heated by attaching a cotton ball that is lit on fire on the opposite tip of the needle. Another is through electro acupuncture where needles are attached with wires that can allow electric current to pass through the needle and reach the meridian point.

With Acupressure

Another school that is similar to reflexology is that of acupressure. The main difference between acupressure with reflexology is that reflexology is primarily centered on the feet, hands and face. On the other hand, acupressure can cover the entire body. You may not know it but you may have already experienced one or another form of acupressure. Some of the more popular spa services, like Shiatsu or Thai massages derive their techniques primarily from acupressure principles.

Techniques are also similar to reflexology techniques, such as thumb walking, using sticks or knuckles. However in acupressure there are other methods being used such as stretching and bending. Still, meridian points are the focus of the acupressure but the massage will involve almost every part of the body. The goal is also removing the blockages that prevent the smooth flow of energy into the vital organs of the body. Of particular interest in the field of acupressure is the balancing of this energy, such as the yin and yang concepts.

Similar to reflexology and acupuncture, the intended effect is to provide relief from pain, reduce tension in the muscles, maintain proper circulation and of course, encourage relaxation. However, in acupressure, there are other health objectives that can be attained, from emotional pains, better sex, addictions and even aesthetic benefits.

Other Complementary Techniques

Aside from acupressure and acupuncture, there are other methods that are done as a complement to reflexology sessions. Moxibustion is the use of several pieces of moxa leaves, which are wrapped into a cone shape and laid near on top of a meridian point. It is then burned sometimes, even directly to create a blister or indirectly such as having a layer in between the moxa cone and the skin.

Another technique is called cupping. In this technique glass bottles are placed on key areas in the body, before they are laid down a match or a lighter is lit inside the bottle and then immediately laid on the skin. When this is done, oxygen is burned and a momentary vacuum is achieved, this creates a suction effect that pulls a certain portion of the skin into the bottle. The suction effect is meant to improve circulation.

Making use of the meridian points again is sonopuncture. Instead of pressure made by the fingers as with acupressure or reflexology or by needles as with acupuncture, sound is used. A tuning fork or a beam of sound is sent directly to the meridian point in question to stimulate the point.

Another technique that is gaining popularity today is of the manipulation of the meridians in the ear. Similar to the meridian points in the hands and feet that correspond to specific organs in the body, the ear is also a microcosm of meridian points that covers most if not all parts of the body. From the spinal cord that can be influenced via the outermost ridge of the ear to the heart that is just outside the ear canal, the ear reflexology is another option for you. Using the ear reflexology chart, acupuncturists also apply a specialty on ear acupuncture.

For a do-it-yourself ear reflexology session, you can start by referring to this chart:

Bryan Thompson

(http://www.handreflexologycharts.com/Reflexology/ear-
reflexology-charts.htm).

Next, you need to bring yourself to a relaxed mood or environment, such as inside a quiet room or on a day when you have a relatively free schedule. Make yourself comfortable by sitting on a chair. If you have long hair that obstructs access to your ear, tie it down first.

Begin with the outer lobes of your ears, start with the right and then the left. Apply gentle pressure by pinching and then pulling down. Next, use your index finger to trace the outer edges from the upper to the lower tip, until you circle the entire ear. Do this for a minute. As you are tracing your ears and gently putting pressure, be on the lookout for any areas that you feel pain or are sensitive to the touch. Make a mental note when you press and you feel from pain from it.

Next repeat the tracing of the edges but this time spend around 5 seconds while exerting pressure. Once you are done move to the next spot until you cover inch of your ear. Try to put pressure on the inner areas of your ear. If your forefinger is too large to reach it, use a cotton bud or any thin stick with a curved or blunt tip that you can use. This is similar to the principle of wooden sticks pressed against the foot in foot reflexology.

Now when you are done with both ears, you can review the sensitive areas that you have encountered during the first steps of your ear reflex session. Now, use the chart to identify which organ the sensitive area corresponds too. You can use this technique as a way of targeting future reflex sessions or deciding on other health choices. Take note, ear acupressure and acupuncture are also available treatments that are related to the ear.

Bryan Thompson

Chapter 12

Selecting Reflexologists

While reflexology can truly be administered by yourself and even at the comfort of your own home, there are still cases that you may require or prefer the assistance of a professional. This is especially necessary for beginners who want to have a firsthand experience of the art so they can do it by themselves on the next sessions. Selecting reflexologists is an important task since you are basically entrusting the care of your body to another person. This is why you need to pay particular attention to your choice.

Bryan Thompson

Local & Online Resources

Your first step in finding and selecting your reflexologists can be done in the comforts of your home. There are three important websites that you can visit to start your search. The first is the American Reflexology Certification Board or the ARCB. This is the board in charge of certifying reflexologists who meet the highest standards of the technique. Rigorous exams are applied to those wishing to reflexologists who wish to be certified. These exams are in turn recognized by local and state governments. A reflexologist with this certification is a mark of not only expertise but also of ethics. A useful tool in the website is the Find a Reflexologist tool that allows you to find a professional and registered reflexologist in terms of location. To visit ARCB, go to http://www.arcb.net/.

Your next online resource for finding a reflexologist is the Reflexology Association of America or the RAA. This is the association of all professionally registered reflexologists in the country. If the ARCB is the certifying body, then RAA is the association that pools them all together. Again you can use the Search Directory to find a list of closest reflexologists that are members of this association. The RAA requires a minimum of 300 hours of training with more than half of those hours received from classroom environments. To visit RAA, go to: http://reflexology-usa.org/.

Finally and more a specific set of searches, you can visit Professional Reflexology Association of your state. For example, if you are from California, you will have the Reflexology Association of California or RAC. If you are from Nevada, then it is the Nevada Reflexology Organization or NRO. Each of these associations can give you referrals to their members within the states or even those from abroad. This website (http://www.holisticwebworks.com/Reflexology-Associations.htm) offers a directory of major associations spread across the US.

Bryan Thompson

Aside from online resources, you can also look your nearest wellness centers or alternative health clinics that will surely be manned by resident registered reflexologists. The more your chosen reflexologists is recognized by these professional organization, the better are your chances for receiving sessions that are both effective and within standards.

Background Check & Referral

Once you have shortlisted your potential choices for a reflexologists, it is important to conduct due diligence. Just as you would ask for background information or referrals from a doctor that you plan on consulting, you also need to do the same step for your reflexologists. Due the various kinds of training on reflexology, including guides similar to this one, it is also necessary to know the extent of the education and experience of your shortlisted reflexologist before making the final choice. While both beginner and expert reflexologist may be familiar with the locations of the meridian points and their corresponding

102

organs, the mark of an advanced reflexologist can be differentiated with his sensitivity to his fingers. Experts have the almost instinctual ability to determine the pressure needed that is just the right balance between gentle but firm and effective pressure.

For other ways to judge the qualification of your shortlisted reflexologists, you can ask for referrals. Ask family, friends and colleagues if they know someone whom they can recommend. While you are asking, investigate what makes them different from other reflexologists. You can also ask other health professionals for recommendations. However, at the end of the day, it is still up to you to determine which reflexologist is best for you.

Remember, reflexology is not a science. This means that though reflexologists may have studied in the same school or may have had the same number of experience as with other reflexologists, he may not be able to produce the objective that you want. Each patient has a unique health profile. This goes the same with reflexologists, he may have received standard teachings but over time, he will develop his own style and upgrade his lessons.

Average Cost

Once you have verified that your shortlisted reflexologists is professional certified or a member of a reflexology association, then you final criteria can be the cost of the professional fee. There is no standard cost on how much a reflexologist can charge for his services. On the average, around $60 to $65 is charged for a session, with the lowest reported to be $35 and the highest to be $100 as of the latest 2015 survey. Tips are also customary but not required. Consider not only the qualifications of your chosen reflexologist but also their affordability to your current financial situation. On a related topic to finances, reflexologists have salary rates almost similar to massage therapist, which is around upwards of $35,000 annual.

Chapter 13

Reflexology Session Expectations

When you have selected reflexologist, it is best to have an idea of what to expect during the session so that you will feel more comfortable, prepared and confident on the session itself. One of the many reasons why people hesitate in trying reflexology is because of the many misconceptions around the sessions. For example, some people believe that during a reflex session, you will be required to undress totally. Some also think that reflexology places are unsanitary or fly by night venues and practitioners.

The reality is wellness centers, which are sanitary and well equipped alternative health clinics, almost look exactly the same as a Western style clinic looks like. There will be a receptionist in the front, a waiting area, open and private areas for the session proper. Since reflexology only involves the feet, the hands and sometimes the face and the ears, there is no need to undress fully. To prepare, you need to come in comfortable clothing and have eaten no meals 2 hours prior to your session. Sandals and slippers are best so that you can easily remove and put them back on after a session. Most reflexology clinics offer foot basins to wash your feet before the session.

Consultation

Just as with a traditional clinic, a reflexology session begins with a consultation. You will immediately know that you are with a professional if he begins with taking your medical history or any other medical information before going straight to the reflex session. Make sure to be as specific as you can with the purpose of your visit. Is it a specific issue that you are aware of or do you have symptoms with causes that elude you? Is your visit more for relaxation or for stimulation of the reflex points? Do you have any medical conditions that you want to address or avoid? Do you have a history of illnesses, prior hospitalization, current medications, and acute or chronic health problems? Aside from taking your vital statistics such as weight, blood pressure etc, and your reflexologist will ask these questions so he can have a better idea on the best and appropriate treatment for you.

Treatment

After the consultation, the treatment process will take place. This time the reflexologist will ask you to sit in a comfortable chair or lie down for better access of your feet. He will most probably ask you to wash your feet before starting. He will then begin by inspecting and touching the area on your feet or hands that correspond to your session objective. At first, he will make light pressure on the area and ask you for your reaction, whether the pressure is tolerable or painful. You are free at any time of the session to ask the reflexologist to lighten the pressure or to stop entirely. A session will average from 30 to 90 minutes. It will be common that the session area will have soft light, aromatic with incense or diffusers and even calming music in the background.

Oils, Powders & Other Supplies

Most of the time, the reflexologist will be using oil or talc powder to reduce friction during the session. If you feel uncomfortable with any of these supplies, you can bring your own and have your reflexologist use it. Usually, oil will be used in the onset and then when the session is done, it will be wiped off with a damp and warm towel. Ordinary talc powder will then be used to remove the sticky feeling of the oil.

Depending on the treatment and also upon your consent, your reflexology session can also include other techniques that belong to its complementary array. For example, if your condition is best addressed with acupressure or applying pressure on not just the feet but also other parts of the body, like the legs or the back, then this may be used. If the reflexologist is also proficient in moxibustion or cupping then you can also have this within the session proper. Warm bags, heated stones, moxi cones are also some of the options that can be presented and recommended to you. Again, you are free to refuse these complementary techniques.

Post Session Effects

Due to the detoxifying effect of the massages, a glass of water, tea or any warm drink is almost always offered to you. It is best to take these drinks as it will help your body flush out whatever toxins were released during the session. If you are hesitant in taking the drinks, make sure to bring a water bottle with you so you can drink as soon as the session is complete.

It is important to manage your expectations after the session. No legitimate reflexologist will claim or guarantee that your desired effects will be felt as soon as the session ends. Sometimes it will take several months or a few years before the total effect of reflexology sessions is felt and the overall goal is achieved. You will most probably be asked to return for another session either after a couple of weeks or a month.

You need to remain patient and keep the course on your therapies. To track your progress, you can create baseline information before you even started with the reflexology session. As you progress through the sessions, monitor your baseline and see how it changes. If there are incremental but positive changes, then you are on the right track. If there are no changes or even negative changes as you progress, then inform your reflexologist right away so you can work on adjusting your sessions.

Chapter 14

Limitations for Reflexology

Despite reflexology being an alternative and non-invasive health practice, there are still specific situations that will contraindicate its use. Make no mistake that reflexology is safe but even some reflexologists will caution you on undergoing sessions when you have specific characteristics or situations.

Contraindications

Pregnant women, especially those during in their first and second month of pregnancy, are generally discouraged to receive reflexology. If needed the meridian points that are associated with the reproductive organs, such as the ovaries and the uterus are either lightly stimulated or not pressed at all. There is also a risk of causing unwanted contractions which can cause pre term childbirth.

For those with fractures, wounds, arthritis or other similar illnesses that affect the feet or the hand, reflexology is automatically contraindicated. For example, if you have a fracture on your hands, then a good alternative is to use foot reflexology.

Those who are prone to develop blood clots or have the presence of floating blood clots in the arteries are also discouraged to undergo reflexology sessions. These blood clots are dangerous when they reach the brain or the heart. When they are dislodged or allowed to move further because of the circulation that is improved by reflexology, then the risk far outweighs the benefit of having the session.

Other illnesses that may prevent you from receiving reflexology include skin diseases, especially communicable types such as chicken pox, those under the influence of alcohol and drugs, varicose veins and bruises, early days of menses, scars from an operation, hormonal implants and sunburn.

Most reflexologists, who are made aware that their patients have present medical issues usually, require a written consent or clearance for the patient's doctor to undergo the session. Be sure to secure these documents prior to your session. Some medical illnesses that require this consent include cancer, epilepsy, asthma, edema, kidney infections, recent operations, sciatica and cardiovascular conditions. Make sure that you are either cleared by your doctor or limit or avoid reflexology sessions when you have any one of these issues. While there are absolute contraindications, then there are also diseases that can be worked around on depending on the severity and the expertise of the reflexologist. For example, hypertension and diabetes can be studied thoroughly so that reflexology can still be done without endangering the patient. Be as transparent as you can with your reflexologist so you can both make informed decisions on your sessions.

Diagnoses

Reflexologists are also not permitted to provide diagnosis of medical conditions. Even if a meridian point is discovered to be tender or painful and it relates to a particular body organ, the reflexologist is still not allowed to declare a specific medical illness or term that can point out the sickness. Diagnosis implies the identification of a current condition that is present and may persist for longer periods of time. In reflexology, it can minimize the guesswork of puzzling medical conditions that may be given light through the meridian points or a general session.

Reflexology does not claim to provide cure to sickness. Instead, it is a holistic treatment that attempts to address not only the physical but also the mental and spiritual needs of a person. Since it is not a science, it does not claim to be appropriate or effective for everybody. Some patients feel no change after a series of sessions while some report improvements after different durations.

Onset & Duration of Effect

Reflexology sessions, like with traditional or Western medicine, builds on its cumulative effects. As your meridian points are stimulated and as your energy flows smoother with every other session, you will feel the relief. Your reflexologist will give you an approximate timeframe of the interval of your sessions and the duration before noticeable effects are felt.

Also, you are discouraged to have reflexology sessions in rapid successions, such as daily or more than once a week. Controlled stimulation is good for the meridian points and the entire body but when you perform or receive repeated stimulation, your body may experience an overload, which can cause or worsen medical issues. Take note that this is not just for reflexology, if you are also undergoing acupressure or acupuncture or any other stimulating massage techniques, then you need to consider them in scheduling the intervals.

Also it is important to note that reflexology is not a cure-all set of techniques. You cannot ignore other positive health practices just because you are undergoing reflexology sessions. For example, if you are experiencing weight control and you are having reflexology to address it; this does not mean that you can ignore your diet. Remember, reflexology is not meant to be a substitute for any traditional or alternative form of health intervention that you are currently undergoing. It is meant to augment their effects with the goal of total well-being. Also, if you are taking any medications or medical treatment, consult your physician on your decision to use reflexology.

Bryan Thompson

Chapter 15

Further Studies

This book represents only the tip of the reflexology iceberg. The world of reflexology is large and no book can claim to possess all information about reflexology. Once you have read this book, experience will take over as your teacher. No book can compare to the lessons brought about my practical and real life applications of reflexology. Of course, creating a solid foundation to which you can build on your passion or decision to pursue reflexology can also be made possible by doing further studies.

Bryan Thompson

Reflexology is constantly being developed but it is does not stop from updating itself with the latest trends and studies that can provide not only the techniques but also the principles, theories and ideas that help reflexologists update their knowledge base. If you are interested in further studies, then you enroll in basic workshops that can last for a few weekends to a few weeks to full blown classes with their own curricula.

Classes

If you intend to purse your studies, then you have to be very wary of choosing your reflexology school or your instructor. You need to be sure that your teacher or school is a legitimate entity that is authorized to teach the techniques. Each school offers a wide range of lessons or classes to choose from, such as the basic hand and foot reflexology techniques. Classes will include discussions on ear reflexology, zone therapy, acupressure, hot stone reflex, acupressure and other basic but complementary techniques. The standard curriculum will start with an overview of the history of

120

reflexology, the difference between Western and Eastern reflexology, human physiology and anatomy, pathology in general and in the feet, ethics and then the clinical phase of the study.

Specializations

After progressing through the basics, which includes classroom and field exposures, you can take part of advanced classes that are more specialized such as Thai reflexology, preventive care, restorative techniques and others. For a list of schools within your state, go here: http://www.reflexologyschools.org/reflexology-schools/american-reflexology-schools/. On the other, if you have the desire but not the time to attend classes, then online classes that are recognized by certifying boards can be a welcome substitute. From watching lecture videos or reading textbooks to practicum sessions involving more than 120 hours of real work, which you need to record for the certifiers review to the final certification exam, these are all the steps needed of an online student.

Certifications

Although certification is not required to practice reflexology, most reflexologists are pursing certification to prove their credibility and increase their marketability to clients. If you are interested in bringing your reflexology from more than just a hobby but a passion or even a business in itself, you can pursue certification. The American Reflexology Certification or ARCB is in charge of certifying aspiring professionally registered reflexologists. There is a requirement of at least 30 hours of hand and 110 hours of foot training to be eligible to attend the class.

On the other hand, the Reflexology Certification Board or the RCB offers certifications to 3 levels of expertise. The most basic level is the Reflexology Practitioner or the RP. The next level is the Certified Reflexologist and the final level is the Master

Reflexologist or MR. Finally another certification the ACARET Accreditation Credentialing is a certificate that proves that you have enough expertise not only to practice but also to teach reflexology. This certificate requires a minimum of 500 hours of study, plus exams.

Remember, learning reflexology even the basic techniques discussed in this books cannot be done overnight. Often you will need charts, supplies and other materials to help you experience being the giving end of the massage. Remember to be patient in studying the techniques. Start with the simplest of techniques, such as applying pressure on a specific meridian part. When you have become an expert with the basic techniques, then you can go further with the more advanced ones.

Bryan Thompson

Conclusion

The principles and techniques listed above are only the tip of the iceberg. Aside from the feet and hands, there are other reflex zones that you can take advantage of during your sessions. Some of the known but still effective reflex zones can be found in the face and the lobes of your ears. The applications of reflexology are wide and broad. I hope this book was able to provide you with a working knowledge of reflexology.

Remember, reflexology is only one of the many therapies you can do for yourself but do not substitute it for any medicine or intervention that your doctor has already prescribed for you. Reflexology is meant to augment and not to replace these prescriptions. Consult your doctor and reflexologist if you intend to rely on the art for your illnesses.

Whether you use reflexology to reduce symptoms, heal illnesses or relax, practicing these techniques will be one of the best decisions you can make for your health and well-being.

Of course, as with any other form of treatment or medicine, the benefits of reflexology do not happen overnight. Often, you need several months and a few years to experience its positive effects on your body. This only means that you need to start as soon as you can, the earlier you start, the sooner you experience the full benefits of reflexology.

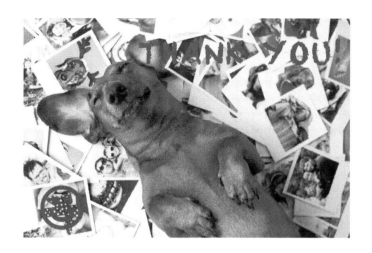

I hope that you are able to find more value in your life through the information resonating inside this book. I do my best to provide content that is accurate, uplifting, and valuable to the reader. If you have any <u>constructive feedback</u> that you would like to offer, or feel like the content in my book can be <u>improved</u> in any way, please feel free to contact me at:

<u>faithinknowledge@bookenthuziast.com</u>

Or go to: **<u>http://amzn.to/1MpekMx</u>**

Bryan Thompson

PREVIEW: YOGA FOR BEGINNERS

Chapter 1 – Relaxing Your Body

"Exercises are like prose, whereas yoga is the poetry of movements. Once you understand the grammar of yoga; you can write your poetry of movements." – Amit Ray

Amit Ray was correct in his assertion that yoga is poetry of movements. In the initial stages of wanting to practice yoga, you may have many misconceptions. For example, you could have seen videos of people who are advanced in the art of yoga and you may mistakenly believe that yoga involves tying yourself up in knots. In fact, yoga is the opposite and unties those knots, letting you become more conscious of your body's needs and your spiritual self. Of course, advanced students can go to extremes in the movements that they perform. Thinking of advanced poets, they can also write epic poems, but you wouldn't expect to do this the first time that you try to write a poem, so don't expect the understand all the nuances before you learn the basics.

One of the main principles of yoga is knowing your body and being comfortable with who you are. The initial exercises in this book are all about relaxation. This is very purposeful. With the kind of lifestyles that people live in this day and age, the chances are that you are stressed, that your body is also stressed and that your mind/body connection isn't that developed. People in today's world are so influenced by pressures laid upon them by modern society that they forget the basics and no longer know how to relax. Relaxation makes you comfortable with your body and is the basic exercise that is used to ease people into their yoga experience.

To learn to relax your body, you need no special equipment, although a yoga mat is always helpful. If you don't have a yoga mat, perhaps a rug or camping mattress will be suitable. These are very thin, roll up mattresses that people use on the beach and are relatively cheap, whereas yoga mats may require more of an investment.

It's helpful to know that relaxation exercises will differ dependent upon age. Age makes the body differ in flexibility. A young person will be much more flexible than someone who is older and thus, there are adjustments made to the relaxation process dependent upon your age and current health.

If you are doing yoga on your own, then you do need to choose somewhere where outside influence will not interrupt your flow of thought. If you have the TV on, turn it off. The idea of the relaxation exercise routine is to concentrate on what you are doing and that's vital to success.

Relaxation exercises

You will need to lie on your back on your yoga mat or equivalent and usually the head is flat on the mat. However, if you are a little older and have experienced neck problems, use a small cushion for your head though once you have become accustomed to exercises, you can remove this. For the time being, it's safer to support your neck. Younger people won't need this as they have much more flexibility.

Breathing correctly

Breathing forms part of yoga exercise. Many people get lazy about their breathing and breath through the mouth all of the time. For correct breathing practice and for the purpose of relaxation, students are asked to breathe in through the nose and breathe out through the mouth. If you repeat this up to a dozen times, you are letting your body get used to the lying position and letting the body relax. Try to concentrate on the breathing and feel the air coming into the body and then leaving the body. Breathing out from the abdomen area helps you to relax and following the flow of the breathing is important because you need to blot out all the thoughts of the day and simply concentrate on your breathing.

If you have never practiced this, you will find that it's hard at first to cut out all of the thoughts that you have. With practice, you will find that you are much more capable of doing this.

Relaxing Every Part of Your Body

This is part of the relaxation exercises that takes place after the initial breathing exercise. As you imagine each part of your body, you need to be conscious of that part of the body. For example, starting from the bottom of your body, close your eyes and imagine your toes, tense the muscles in your toes so that you concentrate on that area of your body. Then relax that area of the body and feel it become heavy and totally relaxed.

During this exercise, keep your eyes closed. Work your way up your body, from your toes to your ankles, from your ankles to your

Bryan Thompson

calf, from that area to your knees etc. going through the same

process of tensing and then relaxing the area

For more information, go to: http://amzn.to/1bA7Jym

Printed in Great Britain
by Amazon

32828284R00077